The Information in this book is to prompt you to explore your health with your Dr and is not given as expert advice. Please contact your Family Dr. or other healthcare provider for more information.

ISBN 978-1-7777068-0-7
First Edition 2021 - Paperback
Authored by Gretchen Theakston
Cover graphics by Eugene McGrath

Healthy you!

Vitamins, who knew?

By

G L Theakston

<u>ABOUT THE AUTHOR</u>

Gretchen Theakston resides in Toronto Ontario
with her son
and their dog Nanook.
Nurse, mother, poet, writer, traveller and dreamer.
She likes reading, walks with the dog in the early
morning and strolling
on the nearby beach.
She has a passion for research and
loves sharing what she finds with others.
Her hope is that you will find this information
of value in your life and journey to health.
If you have questions about the content or
comments
you would like to share feel free to reach out at
emergenceyentrepreneur61@gmail.com
or @emergency_entrepreneur
or https://www.thewitchinme.com

TABLE OF CONTENT

<u>INTRODUCTION</u>

My name is Gretchen Theakston and I am a Nurse in Canada and have been for over 20 years.

I have worked in a wide variety of areas in my profession but eventually ended up in Emergency Medicine.
I must say that I loved it there.
There was always something new to learn and always interesting people passing through.
From one day to the next the people and problems changed and were ever-evolving.
Nursing changed a lot during my career as well, some good, some bad like other professions.

Learning to adapt and being willing to change is a hallmark of this profession and I am grateful to have that perspective.
This Pandemic has left many people reeling about the upheaval and changes constantly being thrown at them.
Every day is a new adventure in uncertainty and some days it is just overwhelming.

So, how can we start to take back control and find small pieces of sanity and routine to help us get through this?

That was the question I had been asking myself as I watched this Pandemic unfold across the world. How did we get here and how do we take care of ourselves and our families?
When is it going to end and what can I do?

Big questions and I was not finding very many good or long-term answers.
So, like a good nurse and a person who loves research, I started looking for answers in the health care professional bodies.
I came across some helpful answers, some not so helpful and I followed along as Dr's discussed symptomatology and treatments.

What to look for, what works, what doesn't, what do the labs say, are there new models that have potential, how long for a vaccine, what is the likelihood that a vaccine will work.
Any new information coming from countries all over the world I was reading.

The one thing that surprised me and the Dr's was,
why are seemingly healthy people getting sick?
What are we missing?
Is there any way to predict who will survive and
who will get sick?

The answer came and it was not good news.
No-one is exempt, no one.
Yes, the elderly are more likely to die as they have
fragile immune systems but no one is exempt.

What to do then?
What were we all missing?
Did anyone have a good answer?
I don't think I have found it but the one thing that
everyone has in common is the food they eat and
the problems with our food chain.
I wasn't surprised by this thought creeping into
my brain.
We have heard about the problems before.
It isn't news.
Eating the way we have become accustomed to
has presented various studies that ask that very
question.

Is our diet contributing to our present state of worldwide behaviours that could be making us more susceptible to this type of Pandemic model and could this happen again?

That was a scary question and the answer was even scarier.
That answer was YES.

I know that many of us have been asking ourselves what we can do to be healthier.
How can we make changes that will benefit us now and in the long run?

That is what I will be discussing.

I am going to cover Vitamins from A - Z.
What they are, how they work for us and where and how to get them, and most importantly, why we need them and how much per day.

How has the government played a part in our diet and how has it affected us?
Has it helped or harmed us?

Is fat really your enemy?
And much more.

I hope you will join me on this discovery I am on.
This Pandemic has given me time to really look at
what we do and what we depend on and how it
affects us daily.
I wanted answers and I found some and I drew
my own conclusions on some as well.
This is not a research paper and this is not my
field of expertise but rest assured that I will be
giving information and citing the papers and
people who I have found give sound advice.

**If you would like to take some of my advice,
please check with your Family Dr. or other
healthcare professionals.
This is not my profession. I am a nurse who
loves discovering new research and sharing it
with others.**

Thank you for your interest.

Gretchen Theakston

<u>LET'S TALK VITAMINS!</u>

I know that many people still don't take vitamins
as part of their health regime.
I get it. It can be difficult to remember to take
them and also to pick them up when you run out

Of course, there is also the question of why
should you take them to begin with.
That is an excellent question and one I hope to
answer as we explore together what they are,
how they work and why we need them in our
society today.

We will start with the A Vitamins and work our
way through them. I am hoping to give you a good
understanding
of Vitamins so you can decide for yourself if they
are right for you.

So, shall we begin?

<u>A Brief History on Vitamins</u>

I have often wondered how and who found out
about vitamins.
It was puzzling to me as I had never come across
this information and never thought to look it up.
I guess because we have all grown up knowing
about vitamins that the question was never of
interest and I am pretty sure that we skipped over
that part in my nursing courses.

This is what I have found in my research.
Physicians once believed that there were only four
things you needed to stay healthy in your life.
Protein, carbohydrates, fats and minerals.
Well, they were partly right as these are the basic
foundations for a balanced diet.
So then why were so many people still getting
sick?

The advent of the germ theory of disease and the
dogma surrounding it had no answer.
So where to look and who was looking?
We do know that some of the main diseases that
could not be identified as related to the germ
theory

were scurvy, rickets, beriberi, pellagra and xerophthalmia and soon enough some clinicians identified them as deficiencies of vitamins rather than disease motivated illnesses due to infection or toxins.

We know that sailors were treated with citrus fruits and told to take them on long voyages to help prevent scurvy so that one had already been addressed but what was causing the problem had still not been identified even though we could curtail the effects.

Kazimierz Funk. a biochemist from Poland, is credited as the first to discover the uses for vitamins which he named vitamines (vit=life, amines=nitrogen/hydrogen-based molecules essential to life) thinking that all the substances he had found came from the same chemical family. He first discovered and studied these in 1911 and released his research paper in 1912.
His findings were duplicated several times over but not all the substances would be considered amines.

The "e" was dropped from vitamines to become what we refer to as vitamins.

We are still discovering more vitamins and their actions on our bodies.
So far, we have much research on 15 but the work continues, as it should.

We have pretty much eliminated many of the vitamin deficiency illnesses that used to plague us but we are not out of the woods yet.
We also have people who suffer toxicity from the overuse of vitamins as well as some remaining deficiencies and this is why many companies put vitamins in their foods.

The question is, are they effective in our foods as additives or should we be getting them another way?

Are supplements effective and if not why?

Should we be taking vitamins daily and will they help our overall health?

Can we get the recommended dosage of vitamins strictly from our food sources?

All great questions that I am going to answer for you. Once you have the information I have found you can do more research on your own and discuss it with your Family Doctor or other health care worker.

**I am not a physician or a professional in this area
and I am only giving you information that I have found helpful for myself.**

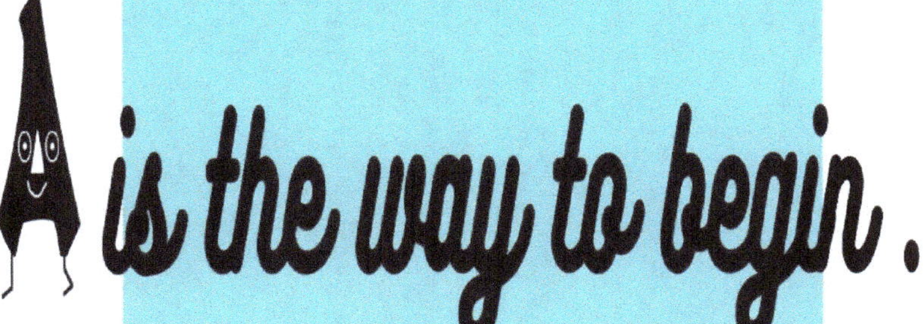

A is the way to begin.

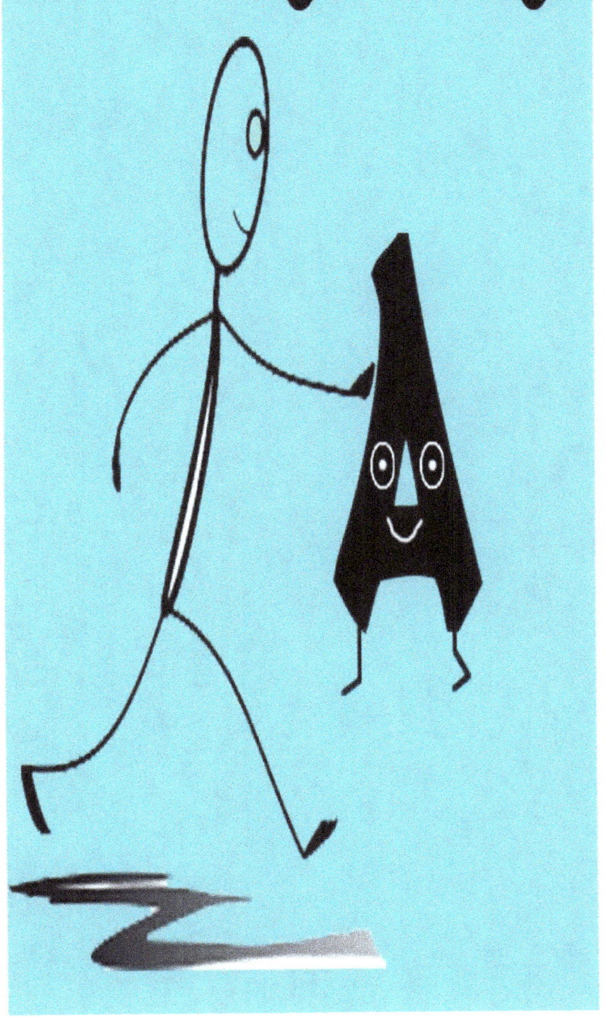

Vitamin A

Vitamin A is quite the powerhouse for our bodies.
From the time we are in the womb and throughout
our life, this vitamin is constantly at work.
Never a day off for this lovely vitamin.
So what does it do and how does it do it?

Vitamin A is integral to the overall working of our
bodies.
It helps keep our immune system healthy and up
to par.
It takes care of all our mucus membranes, and we
have quite a few of them.
It looks after our eyes, our skin and our hair to
keep them healthy and robust.
It also helps us maintain healthy organs, our teeth
and is vital in the womb for proper fetal
development and growth.

It may help in
lowering the risk of some cancers, reduce the
effects of acne and protect your eyes from night
blindness and age-related decline.

Wow, that is a lot of work for one Vitamin!

So how does it work and how do we make sure we get enough to keep it working at an optimum level?

So happy you asked.

Vitamin A is considered a generic term as it covers a group of fat-soluble compounds that our bodies use daily.
Vitamin A compounds can be found in both plant and animal products.
This is where a balanced diet comes in handy.

The active form of Vitamin A (preformed Vitamin A) can be used immediately.
We get it from eating meat, chicken, fish, dairy etc which include the compounds retinol, retinal and retinoic acid.
Because they are easily obtained through eating a balanced diet our body uses it immediately so it does not have to go through any conversion to be used.

The other part of the Vitamin A compound that we need is called Provitamin A carotenoids.

These are the inactive form of vitamin A and are found in plants.
They are called beta-carotene, alpha-carotene and beta-cryptoxanthin.

The above three compounds need to be converted by our body to be activated.
This conversion mostly takes place in the small intestine.

Because this vitamin is often stored in the liver, toxicity can occur.
Most of our vitamin A can be obtained through a balanced diet however, those who are vegan do need to have this vitamin checked occasionally to ensure their vitamin A is maintained at an optimum level.
The standard male dose is 900mcg/day and the female dose is 700mcg/day

So there you have it.
One powerful Vitamin out of the way.
A balanced diet will usually provide all that
you need of this spectacular Vitamin!

**Please make sure you check with your Dr.
before taking this Vitamin.
Most people do not require it as they get plenty
in their diet.**

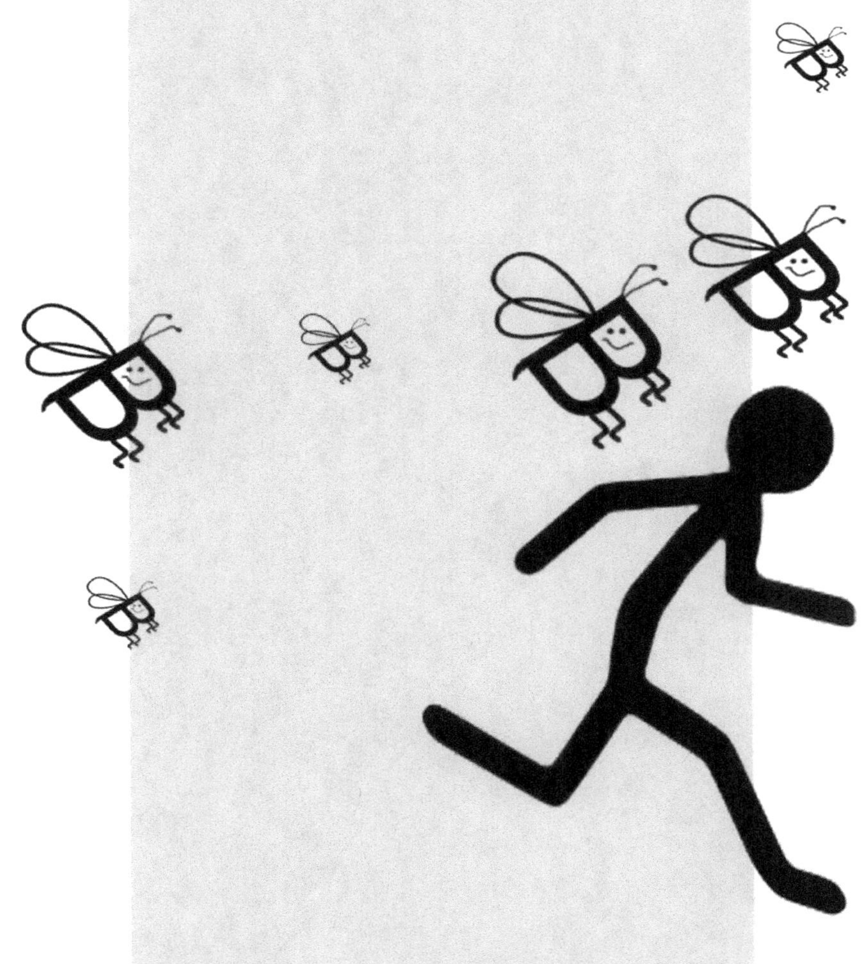

Here come the Bs!

<u>HERE COME THE B'S</u>

Most people know some of these Vitamins as they are listed on the side of many of the products that we eat.
You may not know they are B Vitamins and that's why I wanted to talk about them
Most B Vitamins come as a B-Complex Vitamin and that is how they are generally marketed.
I would like to give you information about all the B Vitamins and how they help us,
First thing you need to know is that they are a water-based Vitamin which means they don't build up in the body and we need to have them in our diet on an ongoing basis.

<u>The B Vitamins are:</u>

B1- Thiamine
B2 -Riboflavin
B3 - Niacin
B5 - Pantothenic Acid
B6 - Pyridoxine
B7 - Biotin
B9 - Folate
B12 -Cobalamin

You may be unfamiliar with some of the names but others I am sure are familiar.

We get most of these Vitamins eating dark leafy greens, brown rice, barley, millet, eggs, milk and milk products, meat, poultry, beans, lentils, sunflower seeds, almonds, citrus fruits, avocados, bananas and the list continues.

With a balanced diet, most of our B Vitamins are consumed daily so this particular Vitamin may not be necessary for your diet.
There are some exceptions and I will be discussing them in this chapter

Let's start with Vitamin B12.
All the B Vitamins are important in our diet but this one can make a critical difference in our lives when we do not get enough.

Here is why.
Vitamin B12 deficiency can result in many health concerns that should be taking you to see your family Dr.

Here are some of the symptoms to look for

Having a pale yellow tinge to your skin
A red and sore tongue (glossitis)
Changes in the way you walk and move around
Disturbed or changed vision
Depression or irritability
Pins and needles in your extremities (paraesthesia)
Possibly mouth ulcers
Changes in the way you think, feel and behave
A decline in your mental abilities
Loss of memory, understanding and judgement

All of the above symptoms or any combination
should prompt you to seek medical intervention.
The question is, why does this happen and how can
we prevent or slow down these changes as we age?

And I say as we age because that is when they first
become apparent.
So why is that?

Science has told us that as we age the way we absorb certain vitamins can be impaired.

One of those reasons is disturbances in our digestive flora, the stuff that helps us identify and breakdown nutrients and vitamins that we require.
As a result of this our ability to uptake B12 declines.

What can we do about it?

The biggest problem we have is that when we start to see these problems cropping up we are way past the point where we can reverse them.
We can slow down the decline but cannot repair the damage that has already occurred.

When should you start keeping an eye on B12?
Great question and unfortunately that is a huge age range.
I would suggest when you are in your thirties and let me tell you why.
This is the age in our life when pressures from work, our relationships and family really start to put a strain on our bodies.

All of a sudden it feels like our career choice might
not be what we thought it was going to be, maybe you
are thinking of getting married, having children,
buying your first home or even getting a divorce.
It is usually the first time that we notice that our
parents are getting older and what happens when
they do and are we going to be responsible for caring
for them?

So many new stress that we had never considered or
even been concerned about
So what about your own health?
Are you keeping a watch on it?
Are you doing everything you can to stay healthy?
Are you having yearly check-up's with your Dr?
Are you eating properly?
Are you exercising?

All these questions should be important but like most
of the population, it is few and far between who
actually do anything about maintaining their health
during this period.
There is just too much going on that our health is the
thing that gets left behind.

The reasoning?
I'm still young
I have plenty of time
I'm healthy
I feel fine
There is nothing wrong with me so why bother

I have been guilty of a few of these myself so I get it.
Unfortunately, these excuses will not protect us
forever so better sooner is now my motto

The other area where B12 becomes important is
during pregnancy.

Lack of B12 can result in what is called neural tube
defect and is a serious birth defect.
The neural tube is a channel between the brain and
the spinal cord and as you can imagine when this is
underdeveloped serious complication can arise

Although most women get to their Dr as soon as they
realize they are pregnant, having a proper amount of
B12 as part of your daily routine would make more
sense than waiting.

So if you plan to become pregnant or even think that might be in your future I would suggest that B12 would be something to keep an eye on.

The third group that can be affected by B12 deficiency is people who practice a vegetarian or vegan diet.

By the way, I am all for this type of diet and am making my way there myself.

Because both these diets do not contain meat, poultry or fish and often have few if any animal products the source of B12 must come from somewhere else. Not surprisingly most of the other choices mean a large consumption practice which is not practical or sustainable.

Again not bashing either choice just letting you know. So, keeping an eye on B12 as part of your yearly health check-up becomes important for people who choose these diets.

B12 can be supplemented using a Vitamin pill or by monthly injections with your family Dr.
The optimum dose for people over 14 - 2.4mcg daily

Over 50 years of age will require more but please check with your family Dr as this dose is also dependent on individual metabolism as well as medications.

Older adults may be prescribed doses from to 500mcg to 1000mcg or more.

The reason I have spent so much time on just B12 Vitamins is the work that they contribute to our daily well being.

B12 is necessary for proper nerve functioning, red blood cell production, DNA formation and our metabolism.

It is also one of the vitamins that play an important role in keeping our levels of an amino acid called homocysteine in check.
High levels of this amino acid have been linked to some chronic conditions and these are heart disease, stroke and Alzheimer's.

Fatigue and lack of energy regardless of your age could mean a B12 deficiency and possibly anaemia.

When you are young, it is easily treatable but when you are older it is a little tougher.

All right, I think I have covered the highlights of B12. The rest of the B Vitamins are fairly easy to get and maintain.

A diet that is balanced can and does easily meet the needs for there requirement.

If you pick up a loaf of bread from the store and look at the ingredients you will see at least 2 of them mentioned.

Crackers, cereals and other fortified foods also contain at least 2 if not more
Check out your milk and see what vitamins are in your dairy products?

Yup, there as well.
Reading our food labels can tell us a lot, not the whole story but a portion that may be helpful when making decisions for your family.

I have spent a lot of time on B12 simply because of its importance to our health. The other B vitamins have an importance to but the impact of a lack of B12 vitamins carries a more devastating impact to our health than the other B vitamins.

So let's have a look at them.

<u>B1 -Thiamin</u>

This B vitamin, like all B vitamins, is water soluble and essential.
Its job is to help our bodies use carbohydrates as energy.
Glucose metabolism depends on B1 and it also plays a key role in heart function as well as in our nerves and muscles

B1 was the first B vitamin to be discovered and that was in 1897 and then isolated in 1926 and was first made in 1936.
It is used to treat beriberi and Wernicke encephalopathy.
It has been used to treat Maple Syrup urine disease as well as Leigh Syndrome.

<u>B2 - Riboflavin</u>

B2 was first discovered in 1920, it was isolated in 1933 and the first time it was synthesized was 1935.
Its primary functions include the breakdown of carbohydrates, proteins and fats so the body can use them for energy.
It is also critical in cellular respiration which is the use of oxygen by the body.

It can be found in many food sources including almonds, dairy products and milk, mushrooms, eggs and green vegetables to name a few.
Most people get more than enough of this vitamin from eating a well balanced diet.

Because it is a water soluble vitamin it needs to be taken daily.
Most commonly found in whole grains, legumes and some meat and fishes which are all easily obtained in a well balanced diet.

B1 can be taken as an oral supplement and in people with a grave deficiency it can be delivered through injection or intravenously.

Many countries require B2 to be added to some foods as the vitamin can be broken down during the food manufacturing process.

So look on the side of your bread, cereal and corn products and you may very well see it listed as an ingredient or additive.

B2 is most often taken as an oral supplement but can be used as an injection as well.
High doses of this vitamin have been used to treat migraines with some success.

Because it is a water soluble vitamin it is one that we need to include daily in our diet.

<u>B3 - Niacin</u>

Niacin is another one of the B vitamins.

This one can be found in poultry, liver, tuna, mushrooms, peanuts, peas and many other foods found in a well balanced diet.
Your body produces B3 using the amino acid tryptophan which is great.

Although not considered one of the most essential B vitamins, the deficiency of this vitamin can result in symptoms related to pellagra which can include skin inflammation or irritation, weak muscles, and digestive issues.

Pellagra was found to be related to alcoholism and malnutrition.

B3 was in fact first used to help with malnutrition and this deficiency if not corrected can be fatal within 3 years.

B3 also helps in the maintenance of clear healthy skin by preventing sun damage and non-melanoma cancers.

It can be used both orally and topically in the form of nicotinamide.
Your Dr may prescribe this for people who are at risk for skin cancer.

B3 is also helpful in reducing HDL (high density lipids), the bad cholesterol.
It has been shown to reduce lipid development and thus reduce cholesterol.

It is also helpful in protecting the heart by assisting in histamine production which has been shown to

increase circulation as well as the reduction of and development of atherosclerosis.

B3 aids in the reduction of arthritic effects and other joint problems like mild bone and joint pain or osteoarthritis as it has strong anti-inflammatory properties.

It has been known to assist in the recovery and repair of worn down cartilage, strengthen muscles, and relieve and reduce joint and muscle fatigue.

Problems with impotence or ED?
B3 assists in improving circulation and has been known to be helpful with this problem.

The blood flow in the genitals can be improved with the regular use of B3.

A healthy digestive tract is also dependent on B3 by aiding in the production of hydrochloric acid which is our main digestive acid.
It can also provide help in the promotion of a healthy appetite.
Along with the digestive tract B3 also increases energy by providing aid in the conversion of fats, proteins and carbohydrates in the metabolic process and is involved in cellular integrity throughout the whole body.

Vitamin B3 can help with diabetes by delaying onset and by making it easier to control HBA1C (diabetic markers) more efficiently.
Along with diabetic control it is known as being a brain booster.
B3 is used by the body to increase and maintain proper brain function and relieve brain fog and assist in memory.
There is research on the impact of B3 on Alzheimer's and other mental conditions.

Your Family Dr or health care provider would be the best one to talk to as far as your individual needs for this vitamin are concerned.

B5 - Pantothenic Acid

This B vitamin is a powerhouse when it comes to breaking down food for daily use.
It can be found in such foods as organ meat, eggs, brown rice, avocados, chicken and beef.

Often this vitamin is added to foods like cereals, milk products (milk, cheese, yogurt) and is also found in broccoli, oats and many other foods found in a well balanced diet.
It is actually found in all living things but the amount varies in each food source.

How does it help us daily?
This B vitamin is critical in the breakdown of fats and converting food to usable energy.
It helps the liver break down certain toxins and drugs.
It assists in the making of haemoglobin, some neurotransmitters, steroid hormones and cholesterol (good LDL).

Because of the prevalence of B5 in so many food groups, deficiency is rare.
The most common form of deficiency is found in people with long term malnutrition.

A well balanced diet will provide more than sufficient amounts of this vitamin for most people.
Toxicity is rare and has not been seen in healthy people.

This B vitamin comes as part of a B Complex vitamin and your B5 vitamin levels can be checked using a urine sample at your yearly check up.

There has not been an upper limit set for the amount to ingest of this vitamin.

I would check with your Dr before taking this as an individual supplement.

Vitamin B6 - **Pyridoxine**

This B vitamin like all the others is water soluble so needs to be replenished daily.
It can be found in organ meats, avocados, beef, soybeans, spinach, fish, potatoes, seeds and many other foods included in a well balanced diet.

B6 is involved in the metabolism of fat, carbohydrates and proteins. It helps support the creation of neurotransmitters as well as the production of haemoglobin.
In fact B6 helps support the activity of over 100 enzymes in the body.

Brain function depends on adequate amounts of B6 as it helps regulate emotions such as depression through the neurotransmitters like serotonin and dopamine.
It may help in the regulation or reduction in depression, and may also reduce the onset or likelihood of Alzheimer's although that is still an ongoing research area.

We do know that the reduction in B6, particularly in the elderly, may increase the diagnosis of depression, again that study is still ongoing.

It may also play a role in decreasing homocysteine levels which have been linked to depression and other psychiatric issues.

B6 deficiency has been linked to anaemia which is the result of a decrease in blood cell production. Because B6 aides in the production of haemoglobin.

It has been used to treat pregnant women who do not respond well to iron supplements and has shown an improvement with mild symptoms of anaemia.

This vitamin has been shown to be effective in helping reduce cholesterol in patients at risk by decreasing cholesterol production.

It has been known to help with nausea during pregnancy and reduce PMS symptoms like anxiety and irritability.

The inflammatory effects of Rheumatoid Arthritis have responded well to B6 and can be helpful for people who do not respond well to traditional inflammatory medication.

It has not been found to reduce the level of discomfort or pain and has contributed very little to the increase in agility.

There is evidence that living in a city that has a measurable amount of pollution can and does impact our health negatively.
B6 has been shown to help combat some of the effects on the body.

Like all supplements, please consult with your Family Dr or Healthcare Provider before taking any.
Some medications are not compatible with supplement use and can be dangerous to your health.

<u>B7 - Biotin</u>

Once referred to as vitamin H because it was named Haar und Haut, (a German term meaning hair and skin) it is now called vitamin B7 or biotin.

There is no solid research that taking B7 will help you with thinning hair or get stronger nails but the research does continue in this area.

So what does this vitamin do and how do we get it?

B7 needs to be acquired daily as we do not store it.

It can be found in such foods as organ meats, nuts and nut butters, whole grains and cereals, mushrooms, cauliflower and bananas to name a few. A well balanced diet will give you all you need.

Raw or less processed food can give you more B7 than cooked as the process for consumption can reduce the effectiveness of this vitamin.

Enzymes that are involved in the metabolic breakdown of fats, proteins and carbohydrates need this vitamin for energy and function in these processes.

B7 plays a crucial role in initiating the steps for the metabolic process of fatty acid synthesis, gluconeogenesis and the breaking down of amino acids to name a few.

There has been research that does show some help in keeping your skin healthy, your hair stronger and may reduce hair loss as well as thickening the nails to reduce breakage, the studies continue as it is felt the research has not given a definitive answer yet.

B7 has been shown to lessen the impact on the kidneys of Type 1 diabetics and may be helpful for Type 2 diabetics as well.
There has been research to show that B7 is reduced in both types of diabetics.
The research continues but upping your B7 intake would not do any harm as excess will be excreted.

The other use of vitamin B7 that has shown health benefits is in pregnant women.

It helps with the overall health of the mother and as a result helps the growth and development of the fetus.

Please consult with your Family Dr or other health care professional to see if this is one that you need.

Deficiencies are rare with this B vitamin and are usually found in people with specific syndromes and not normally in the general population.

The best way to ensure you are getting an adequate amount of B7 is to eat a well balanced diet.
If you are going to take a B vitamin, take a B complex supplement as that will offer the best way of ensuring that you are getting the recommended amounts.

Again, please consult with your Family Dr or healthcare professional.

B9 - Folate

Finally at the end of the B vitamins and this is an important one.

I am pretty sure that many of you have heard of B9.
You may know it as Folic Acid or Folate.
Both are B vitamins and there is a difference between the two.

Let's look at Folate first.

This is the form of vitamin B9 that is naturally formed and is the generic name of a group of related compounds that have many similar nutritional properties.
The word Folate is derived from a Latin word, folium, meaning leaf.

Appropriate as one of the best ways of getting B9 is through green leafy vegetables.

The conversion of this vitamin takes place in the digestive tract (stomach) where it is converted into 5-MTHF before entering the bloodstream.

Important in the formation of red blood cells, healthy cell growth and function as well as being critical in early pregnancy to decrease possible
brain formation defects and spinal deformation.

A healthy balanced diet that includes dark green leafy vegetables, beans, peas, nuts as well as oranges, lemons, bananas, melons and strawberries.
Vegetarians and vegans definitely have a leg up on this B vitamin!

Folic Acid is the synthetic form of B9 and is used to fortify many foods in our diet.
Most often found in breads and cereals and has in fact been mandated in many countries to be added due to the historical problems of deficiency.

Folic acid plays a crucial role in healthy brain function and has been linked to mental and emotional health.

Folic acid, along with B12, helps in the production of red blood cells and assists with the work of iron in the body.

Unlike Folate, Folic acid converts in the liver or other tissues which results in a slower metabolizing of this B9 vitamin.
Taken in a B complex vitamin supplement results in the increased ability of this vitamin to be metabolized at a quicker rate!

There are ongoing studies of this B vitamin as they relate to heart disease, stroke, dementia, depression and cancer.

The one area that we know it does affect is the reduction of neural tube defects.
Pregnant women should be taking folic acid as a supplement 3 months before pregnancy and throughout the pregnancy.

Please follow your Family Dr.'s or healthcare professionals advice in this area

Wow, I can't believe we are finally through the B vitamins.

I hope you agree that the B vitamins are a critical part of our overall health and how we eat can and does impact this particular vitamin.
So, where is my salad?

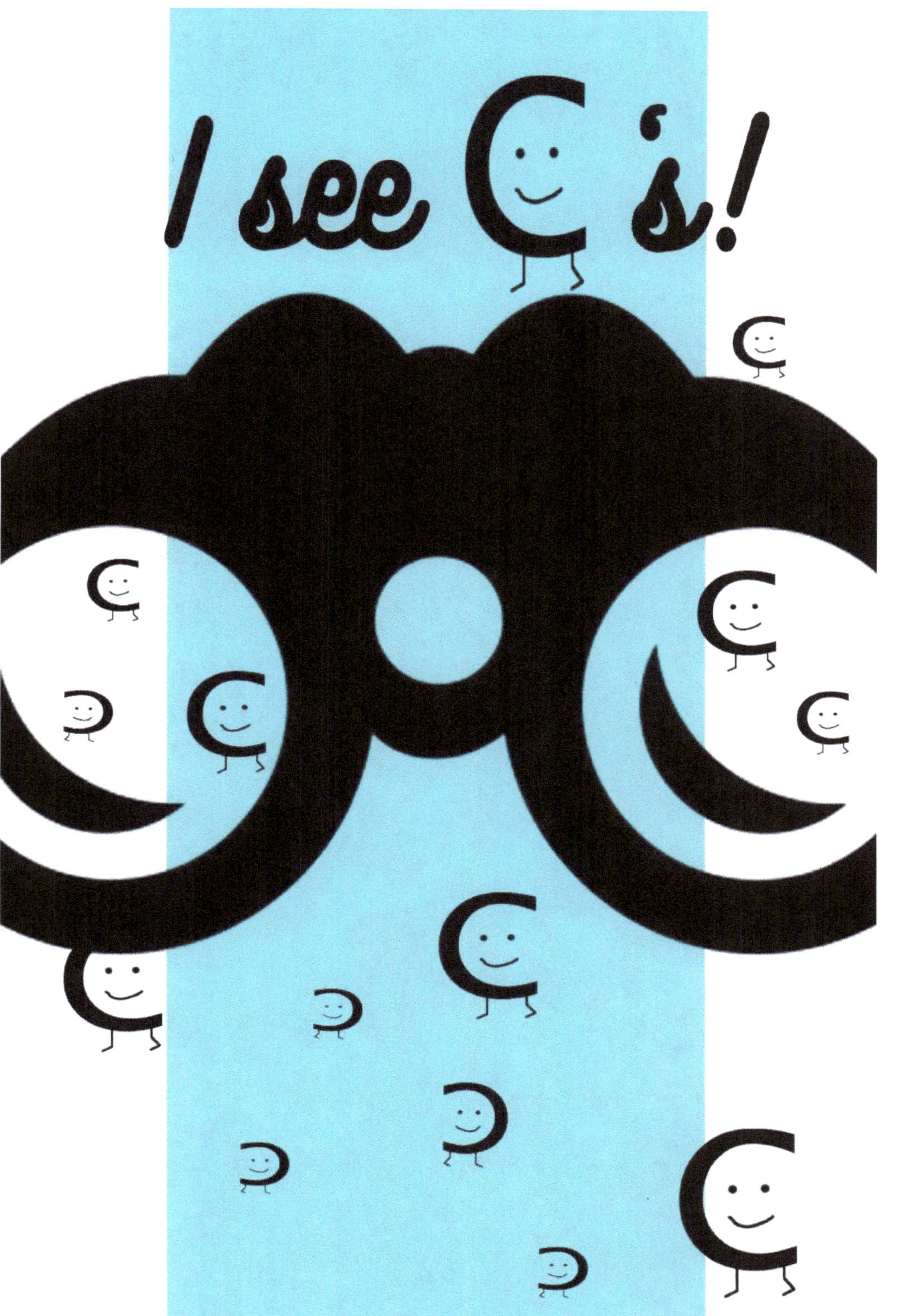
I see C's!

<u>I SEE C'S</u>

Vitamin C, you know it, you love it!
Or do you?
Let's find out what C is all about.

Vitamin C is an essential vitamin and one that we do
not make therefore we need to ingest
it daily in one form or another.
It can be found in many fruits and vegetables like
citrus fruits, Brussel sprouts, potatoes, berries,
tomatoes, peppers, cabbage, spinach and many
others.

It has been suggested that only 10% to 20% of
people get enough vitamin C in their diets so
supplementation is important.
You can safely take up to 2000 mg of vitamin C daily
as that is the upper limit.

However, it is recommended that the daily limit be
500mg, and any excess will simply be excreted.

It's considered one of the safest supplements and one of the most widely prescribed.

So what does it do for us?

Vitamin C is essential in the assistance of numerous enzymatic reactions like the biosynthesis of collagen, carnitine and neuropeptides as well as in the regulation of gene expression.
It helps your body with the formation of blood vessels, cartilage as well as muscle and collagen in bone.
It helps form an important protein that is used to make skin, tendons and ligaments.
It is also a powerful antioxidant and has been shown to assist in the reduction of inflammation.
What other benefits can we derive from taking vitamin C daily?

It may reduce uric acid in the blood thus reducing or eliminating gout.
It has been shown to help with the lowering of blood pressure as it helps to relax the blood vessels.
Excellent for both people with hypertension and those with normal blood pressure.

It protects us from the damage of free radicals and from smoke, second-hand smoke and pollutants. It also protects the integrity of our eyes and our skin so fewer wrinkles.

Diabetics can benefit from a daily intake of vitamin C as their medical condition has been known to leave them in an immune-compromised position.

There are also ongoing studies to determine if a daily vitamin C regime could impact diabetes enough that insulin may stop being the prescribed choice for them.

I am looking forward to hearing more about research and studies in this area.

Research papers have also suggested that allergies can be reduced by high IV injections of vitamin C.

As vitamin C has anti-inflammatory responses and allergies are an inflammatory reaction this research that is ongoing, does have some promise although no definitive research has yet been released.

Low levels of serum vitamin C have been linked to an impaired ability to remember
and to think and several studies have shown that people with dementia do have low levels of serum vitamin C.

It is not yet certain that vitamin C can help in this area but it has been suggested that having adequate serum vitamin C can only help in protecting the brain and any inflammatory reactions it may undergo or be susceptible to. Vitamin C also helps boost our immune system which I am sure is the reason most people take it.

It helps with the absorption of iron which will prevent an iron deficiency.

Vitamin C is also one of the vitamins used in the formation and strengthening of our teeth.
There are studies that have shown that people with serum vitamin C deficiencies who develop pneumonia have had clinical improvements using high dose vitamin C supplementation.

There is more study to be done in this area but the base conclusion is that high dose vitamin C may help in increasing immune function.

Finally, it can help with memory and thinking as we age so keep it handy.

Like all water-soluble vitamins that need to be replaced daily, we do need to eat a well-balanced diet and one rich in vitamin C foods can deliver all the vitamin C that you will require.

Please check with your Family Dr. or other healthcare providers if you have any questions and follow their suggestions,

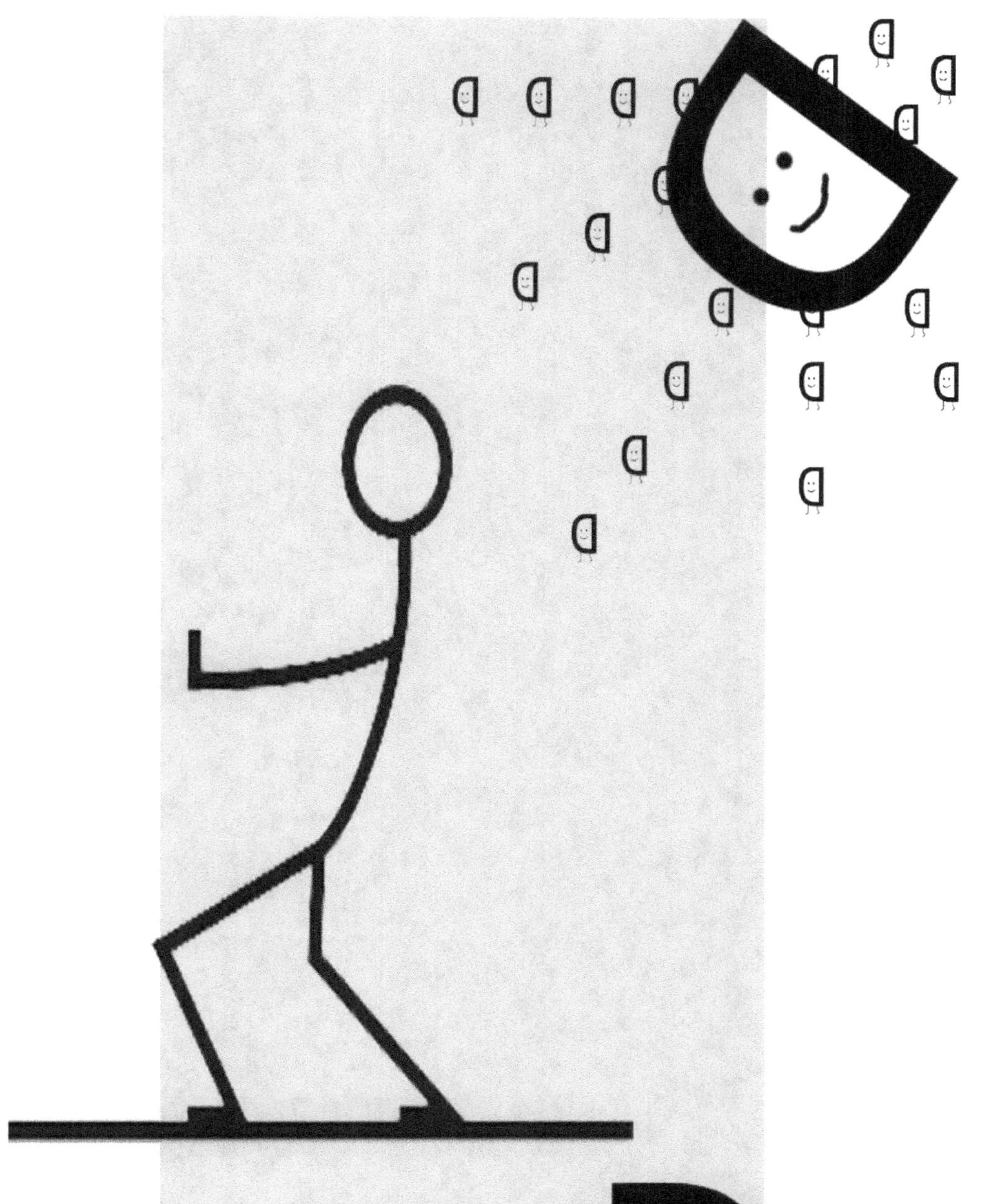
Hello sunny D's!

HELLO SUNNY D'S

Vitamin D

Most people have heard of vitamin D and why it is
referred to as the sunlight vitamin.

You are right, sun exposure is the quickest way to get
vitamin D.
So what does it do for us and how important is it to
our overall health?

Excellent question!
Let's have a closer look at this vitamin.

Vitamin D has two designations, Vitamin D2 and
Vitamin D3.

D3 is the more commonly used variant as it raises
the level of vitamin D in the body significantly faster
than D2 by a factor of 2.

Commonly found in foods such as mushrooms, oily
fish, egg yolks and fish liver oils.

We cannot ingest enough to maintain optimum
levels without the help of sunlight absorption.

Because we often apply a sunscreen that blocks the ability of our skin to absorb this vitamin we find ourselves in a position of having to take it as a supplement year-round.

Living in northern climates or having darker skin does mean that you are at risk of not getting enough vitamin D as it is not something we can produce without sunlight or within our own bodies.

People with darker skin face the same problem and have been found to have significantly lower levels of vitamin D.

It is estimated that 42% of the U.S. population is deficient in vitamin D and that rises to 82% for people with darker skin.
No wonder there has been so much talk about this vitamin lately.

There is a lot of interest in vitamin D right now and the news just keeps getting more and more interesting as the research continues.

We have learnt that there are receptors for this vitamin on almost every cell in your body and that has and is leading to some great research.

We already know that we can prevent rickets (a vitamin D deficiency) in children and can help prevent osteoarthritis as we age.

What we are now learning is that it may be helpful in the reduction of symptoms related to rheumatoid arthritis and the slowing down of the progression of the disease.

The research is ongoing but very promising.

There have been studies that suggest that a deficiency in vitamin D may result in type 2 diabetes, multiple sclerosis, cancer, thyroid problems and high blood pressure.

Some new studies are suggesting that we could delay or help eradicate Alzheimer's disease.

This is exciting news!
Much more study is needed in this area but preliminary studies are hopeful.

We know that vitamin D has some inflammatory properties which is good news for people with autoimmune diseases.

There have also been some preliminary studies on vitamin D and how it relates to Autism.

It has been shown to help with alleviating some of the abnormal social behaviours in people on the autism spectrum.

It does not cure autism, just addresses behaviours.

With all the different research going on I think we are going to be seeing more and more uses for this vitamin.

There are studies going on in the areas of cardiovascular health, cancer, diabetes and longevity.

So what is the optimum dose of vitamin D for adults?

That question varies from study to study as there is no standard for testing bloodwork or for identifying what the optimum levels should be.
Right now most studies agree that adults should be aiming to have 30ng/mL in their bloodwork.

So how do you achieve that?

We cannot get enough in our food even with additives and many people (up to 90% of the population) do not spend enough time outside or they live in areas where sunlight is a seasonal problem, their skin is too dark or they are ageing which also reduces the ability to absorb sunlight.

Taking supplements is in fact the only way to ensure adequate vitamin D is supplied to us each day.

The recommended dosage is anywhere between 200 IU to 2000 IU's so having a discussion with your **Family Dr or other Healthcare provider would be on the to-do list.**

Vitamin D can be taken in both liquid or tablet form and has been proven to be effective in both forms.

Because this is an ever-evolving area of research, more news will be coming to the forefront in the next few years.

Any news that helps us stay healthy longer is always welcome!

Enough about that 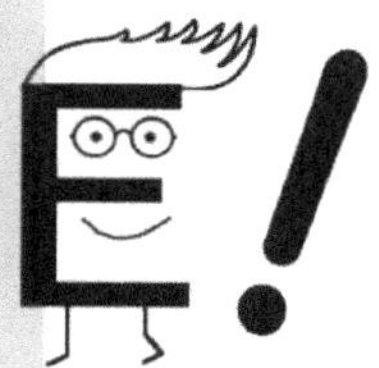!

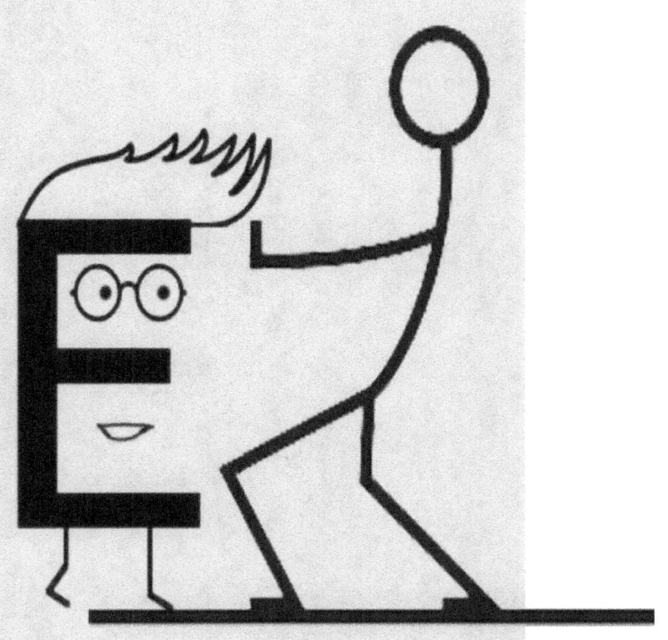

ENOUGH ABOUT THAT E!

Vitamin E

This vitamin has been talked about many times over the years.
You may have heard that if you use it on your skin it will reduce wrinkles and keep your skin looking young.

Is this true or just something beauty companies made up to entice you to invest in their products?

Let's check with science and see what it has to say.

We can get most of our vitamin E from a well-balanced diet which is great news.
Foods that are rich in vitamin E include such processed food as cereal, juice and margarine but there are additives in these products.

How about other foods where it is naturally derived and not an additive?

They include such things as abalone, salmon and other kinds of seafood, broccoli, spinach and other green vegetables, nuts and seeds as well as oils like safflower and sunflower as well as wheat germ.

That is quite a list and gives us lots of options to include it in our diet.

Taking a vitamin E supplement is not necessary unless your Family Dr. or other Healthcare advisor has recommended it.

So what does it do for us?

Vitamin E is an antioxidant and plays a role in reducing free radical damage to our cells.
It also assists in stopping plaque build up in our blood vessels and dilates our blood vessels to ease the movement of blood through our system.
In Vitro studies have shown that it helps with cell expression and metabolic processes.

There are ongoing studies to see if vitamin E can help in the reduction or prevention of free radical damage that may be associated with chronic diseases

Here is the thing about vitamins and our skin, eyes and health.

We do not need added vitamin E as we get enough in our diet and supplementation is not recommended but vitamin C and vitamin E combined may help ease or prevent skin damage from UV light.

The research is ongoing and we do not have a definitive answer yet.
Yes, vitamin E is great for our eyes and helps with some delays in vision loss but that does not require a supplement, just a healthy diet.

Vitamin E and your beauty regime.

Does it hurt or help you?

There has been a lot of new innovation surrounding the use of vitamin E in cosmetics.
It was believed for a long time that there was no evidence of topical application showing any benefits.

How times change!

There is new research showing that new formulations are having some positive effects.
Not definitive yet but certainly moving in that direction.

This is good news for people that are using cosmetics and skin creams daily or other topical applications.
Having vitamin E in these forms as an additive will certainly make them less harmful for daily use.

Even with this promising research most of us do not require added vitamin E as we get enough in our diet and from our own bodies.

This is one vitamin that you should check with your Family Dr. or other Healthcare professional before adding to your list of supplements.

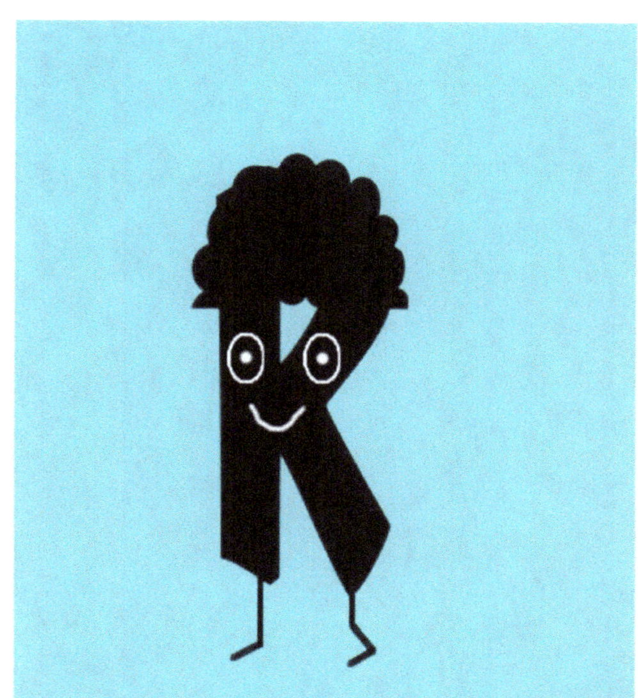

we are nearing the end

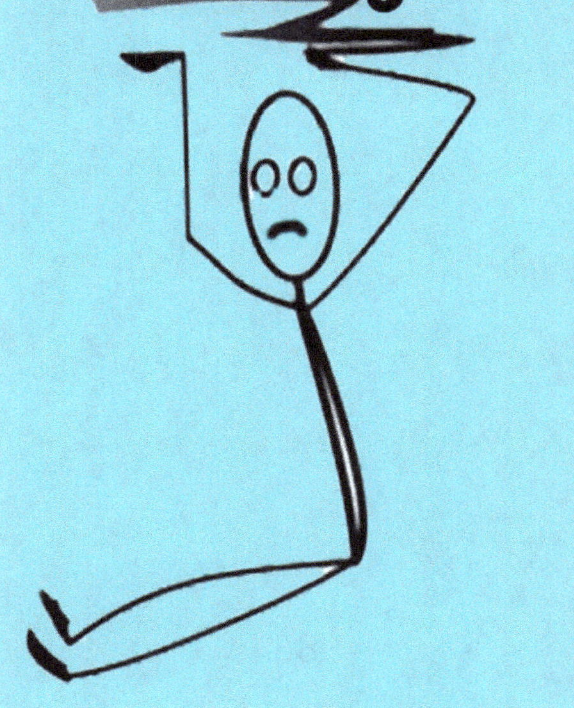

K, WE ARE NEARING THE END

<u>Vitamin K</u>

Here we are at the last vitamin, vitamin K.
This vitamin is the primary reason that our blood
clots but that is not all it does.

It is also concerned with bone health as well as heart
health and helps in the healing of wounds.

There is ongoing research in the area of coronary
disease and if vitamin K would be beneficial in this
area.

There is also research that suggests that having
optimum levels of vitamin K results in less
impairment of brain function over time.

Because vitamin K is readily available in food sources
it is easy for us to maintain optimum levels of this
vitamin by eating a well-balanced diet.

Foods that contain vitamin K are easy to find and add
to our diet.
Kale, broccoli, Brussel sprouts, collard greens, green

onion, pork chops, beef liver and any dark green vegetable to name a few.
The list is long and varied so try a few and have some fun with the choices!

Having a vitamin K deficiency or toxicity is rare in today's societies with the abundant food sources we have available.
A healthy well-balanced diet will certainly keep you on track with this one.

The only time you will have to up your diet rich vitamin K foods is when you are on antibiotics.
Antibiotics are known to reduce the ability of the digestive tract to breakdown and convert vitamin K for our body to use.
This would only become a problem if you had to take antibiotics for long term use.

Babies, upon birth, are given a vitamin K shot as a standard practice as their ability to clot blood is known to be at risk.

**If you are concerned about your vitamin K levels or you are on blood thinners, please consult your Family Dr. or Healthcare professional.
Do not take this vitamin as a supplement unless it has been prescribed.**

AND THAT'S ALL FOLKS, PHEW!

The End

Well, that was quite a journey!
I hope that you have learned something along the
way and are now more connected to your body.
I know I am!

If you are interested in learning more you will find
resources listed that will show you where I
researched and compiled the information from.
There is plenty of reading if you want more in-depth
information.

If I have made errors please feel free to contact me
and let me know.

We are all learning together and I certainly don't
mind being shown where I am wrong.
If you have any questions or you enjoyed the
information and found it helpful, please let me know.

One further bit of information I think I need to be
passing along.

If you are interested in taking supplements please know that not all vitamins are the same.

Research the company that you would like to source your supplements from.
This is a multi-billion dollar industry and not all companies are on the up and up so be aware of who you are working with.

There is plenty of information on the companies available to the public.
Please take advantage of that.
I have looked into many companies but it is not up to me to talk about them.
If you have questions about how to find information please reach out as I would be happy to help.

This is only the beginning and if you have enjoyed it please let me know.

Thank you for coming along on this journey and I hope to see you again!

Gretchen Theakston

RESOURCES

BOOKS

COMMON CURES FOR EVERYDAY AILMENTS
Bottom Line Health

FIGHT BACK WITH FOOD
Reader's Digest

FOOD CURES
Breakthrough NutritionalPrescriptions for
Everything From Colds to Cancer
Reader' Digest

IT STARTS WITH FOOD
Dallas Hartwig &Mellisa Hartwig

PRESCRIPTION FOR NUTRITIONAL HEALING
Fourth Edition
A Practical A-To-Z Reference To Drug-Free Remedies
Using Vitamins, Minerals $ Food Supplements
Phyllis A. Balch, CNC

THE ENCYCLOPEDIA of NATURAL MEDICINE
Third Edition
Michael T. Murray, N.D, and Joseph Pizzorno, N.D.

THE ESSENTIAL GUIDE TO PRESCRIPTION DRUGS
1991
James W. Long, M.D.

THE MERRICK MANUAL OF MEDICAL
INFORMATION
The Home Edition 1997
Robert Berkow, M.D., Mark H. Beers, M.D.,
Robert M. Bogin M.D., Andrew J. Fletcher, M.B., B.
Chir.

THE WORLD'S GREATEST TREASURY OF HEALTH
SECRETS
Bottom Line/Health

WEBSITES

https://www.buckinstitute/vitamins/

https://my.clevelandclinic.org/health/vitamins/

https://facty.com/vitamins/

https://www.hsph.harvard.edu/nutritionsource/vitamins/

https://lpi.oregonstate.edu/mic/vitamins/

https://www.mayoclinic.org/healthy-lifestyle/nutrition-and-healthy-eating/expert-answers/vitamins

https://medshadow.org/vitamins/

https://ods.od.nih.gov/factsheets/vitamins/

https://www.webmd.com/vitamins/

https://10faq.com/vitamins/

ILLUSTRATION AND GRAPHICS

Creatorid'immagine from Noun Project

Eugene McGrath VGS Agency

Kirby Wu from Noun Project

Parkjisun from Noun Project

CONTACT INFORMATION

emergencyentrepreneur61@gmail.com

@emergency_entrepreneur

https://www.thewitchinme.com